Contents

Understanding Carbohydrates

========================

Learn How to Use Them for Health and Weight Loss

RON KNESS

Disclaimer

This publication is for informational purposes only and is not intended as medical advice. Medical advice should always be obtained from a qualified medical professional for any health conditions or symptoms associated with them. It is important to ask a doctor before starting any diet program.

What Are Carbohydrates?

To maintain good health carbohydrates are one of the three main macronutrients we should eat every day; the other two are protein and fat. Carbohydrates support various bodily functions, including providing energy, supporting immune system functions, and blood clotting. In simple terms, carbohydrates are types of sugars converted by the body and uses for energy. Basically there are two types.

Types of Carbohydrates

- Simple Carbohydrates
- Complex Carbohydrates

Simple Carbohydrates

Simple carbohydrates are simple sugars made up of only one or two sugar (saccharide) molecule chains. All simple sugars and starches are converted to glucose in the body with the exception of sugar alcohols and insoluble fiber.

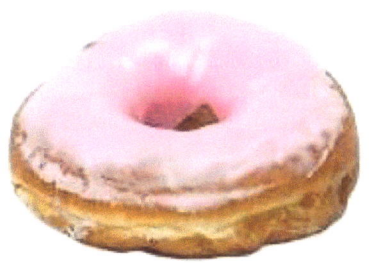

Simple carbohydrates include such foods as:

- Corn syrup
- Baked Goods
- Molasses
- Pizza
- White flour
- Soft drinks
- White bread
- Maple syrup
- Pretzels
- Brown sugar
- Cake
- Candy
- Muffins
- Fruit drinks, natural and artificial
- Cookies
- Fruit sugar (Lactose)
- Chips

- Jellies and jams

- Pastries

- Raw sugar

- Pancakes

- Honey

- Table sugar (Sucrose)

- High fructose corn syrup

However finding sugar in foods is not always easy. In some cases, it can be as simple as reading a nutrition label; in other cases it is more difficult to recognize.

Hidden or not, we should cut back on the amount of foods we eat with the word "sugar" or one of its other names on the label. Greedy food manufacturers are one step ahead of you. They disguise sugar under a wide variety of names. The next time you read a food label and you see any of the phrases listed below, you are really looking at sugar:

- Sucrose

Nutrition Facts

Serving Size 8 oz (227 g/8 oz)
Servings Per Container About 3

Amount Per Serving

Calories 180   Calories from Fat 60

	% Daily Value*
Total Fat 6g	10 %
Saturated Fat 1g	5 %
Trans Fat 0g	
Cholesterol 5mg	2 %
Sodium 75mg	3 %
Total Carbohydrate 26g	9 %
Dietary Fiber 5g	19 %
Sugars 11g	
Protein 8g	

Vitamin A 60 %	•	Vitamin C 70 %
Calcium 8 %	•	Iron 10 %

* Percent Daily Values are based on a 2,000 calorie diet. Your daily values may be higher or lower depending on your calorie needs.

		Calories	2,000	2,500
Total Fat	Less than		65g	80g
Sat Fat	Less than		20g	25g
Cholesterol	Less than		300mg	300mg
Sodium	Less than		2,400mg	2,400mg
Total Carbohydrate			300g	375g
Dietary Fiber			25g	30g

Calories per gram:
Fat 9   •   Carbohydrate 4   •   Protein 4

- Maltose
- Dextrose
- Fructose
- Glucose
- Galactose
- Lactose
- High Fructose Corn Syrup
- Glucose Solids
- Golden Syrup
- Turbinado
- Sorghum Syrup
- Refiner's Syrup
- Ethyl Maltol
- Maple Syrup
- Yellow Sugar
- Agava Nectar
- Cane Juice
- Dehydrated Cane Juice
- Cane Juice Solids
- Cane Juice Crystals
- Dextrin
- Maltodextrin
- Diatase
- Diatastic Malt
- Fruit Juice
- Fruit Juice Concentrate
- Dehydrated Fruit Juice
- Fruit Juice Crystals
- Dextran

- Barley Malt
- Beet Sugar
- Corn Syrup
- Corn Syrup Solids
- Caramel
- Buttered Syrup
- Carob Syrup
- Brown Sugar
- Date Sugar
- Malt Syrup

... and any word on a food label ending in -ose.

According to the website SugarScience.org, and other health authorities, **as much as 74% to 80% of all the packaged foods in your local supermarket contain sugar!** Even foods which brag about having "no high fructose corn syrup" can have dangerously high levels of sugar hidden under some other name.

Complex Carbohydrates

Complex carbohydrates on the other hand are made up of thousands of sugar chains making them "complex". They include such basic foods as starchy vegetables, like corn and potatoes, along with bread, beans, rice, cereals, and grains. Here is a more complete list:

- Brown rice

- Dried fruit

- Raw fruit

- Whole wheat

- Almond flour

- Oat bran

- Bran cereal

- Barley

- Vegetables

- Buckwheat

- Berries

- Cornmeal

- Quinoa

- Oatmeal

- Whole grains

- Wheat germ

- Potatoes

- Rye bread

- Lentils

- Peas

- Hummus

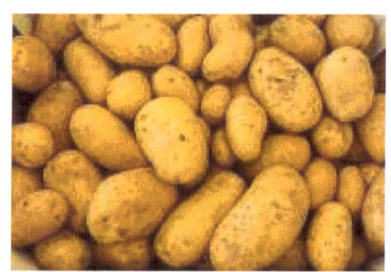

- Beans

- Avocados

- Yams, sweet potatoes

You will notice from this list, as opposed to the simple carbohydrate list, you are looking at a lot of natural fruits, vegetables and whole grains. Most fruits contain a decent amount of natural sugar, but because fruits are high in fiber, that sugar is not as unhealthy for you as processed or refined sugar. Eat more complex carbohydrate foods than simple carbs, and better health is your reward.

How Carbs Work

Of these two, complex carbohydrates are the healthiest, since they also have fiber, nutrients and do not cause blood sugar spikes as simple sugars do. All complex carbohydrates convert to glucose in the body, which is then used as fuel for the cells, brain, and other vital organs. This is why carbohydrates are considered an important part of the human diet.

Because complex carbohydrates are made up of long chains of simple sugars all attached in to one another in various ways, they are too big to be digested by the small intestine in their present state. Therefore, they need to be broken down for absorption into the bloodstream. This takes some time, especially when complex carbs include an ample amount of fiber, like whole grains and brown rice.

Because of the time it takes, glucose increase in the bloodstream is very gradual so that there are no spikes in insulin levels, thus helping to prevent Type 2 diabetes and making sure less sugar turns into fat.

Simple carbohydrates are basically small sugars that are not connected to one another or that have just one connection. These include glucose, fructose, and galactose and do not need to be broken down any further to be absorbed into the body to be used as fuel. So they digest quickly and flood the bloodstream with glucose causing insulin spikes to occur.

Simple Sugars: Fructose And Sucrose

While both are simple sugars, the sugar in fruit is a monosaccharide called fructose, and table sugar is a disaccharide known as sucrose.

Simple sugars aren't as healthy like complex sugars because of the blood sugar spikes they cause. This triggers the release of insulin from the beta cells of the pancreas, which moves the digested sugars into the cells. Leftover sugar is stored as fat, which contributes to weight gain and obesity. Table sugar and anything made with it is considered empty calorie food that typically serves no nutritional purpose for the body. With that said, it is still better than most artificial sweeteners.

While the fructose in fruit is also a simple sugar, it has a natural advantage over table sugar because fruit also provides various nutrients, like antioxidants, minerals, and vitamins that help to reduce cancer, diabetes, and heart disease. Conversely, table sugar has none of these benefits and in fact can actually cause harm to the body beyond weight gain.

It is important to note that eating any type of sugar, especially in large quantities can be harmful, including that which comes from fruit. Typically eating a lot of sugar results in consuming too many calories. Fruit, while nutritious has three times more calories per serving as vegetables.

Simple Carb Foods

Simple sugars are found in any type of processed food product requiring sugar in the recipe. This can include cakes, puddings, pies, cookies, and sugar-containing sodas, among others listed earlier in this book. If you read the food label, it will tell you the amount of carbohydrates in the food as well as the amount of "sugar," which means simple sugars.

Fruit juices also contain simple sugars and no fiber and while juices have a great deal of vitamin C and other healthy ingredients, they are not recommended for those with diabetes or pre-diabetes and for those who are concerned with their bodyweight. The excess sugar in juice just goes to fat.

And quantity of juice is an issue most people don't think about. If you eat an orange, you are getting the juice (and good fiber) from just that one orange.

However, have a normal size glass of orange juice and you are getting the juice from three oranges (and three times the sugar) and in most cases none or very little of the fiber.

Complex Carb Foods

It is a good idea to get your carbohydrates from sources containing complex carbohydrates, especially those with high amounts of fiber. Many naturally low carb foods are healthy and will not cause weight gain when they are a part of a well-balanced diet. Some good foods that contain complex carbohydrates include the following:

- Green vegetables are your best source of carbs as they contain very little impact carbs – the kind that raises blood sugar - and a lot of vitamins, antioxidants, minerals and are high in fiber. For some green vegetables, it takes more calories to break them down, than they contain, making them a negative calorie food and a good choice.
- Brown rice contains a lot of carbs as well as fiber.
- Whole grain bread products that contain real whole grains and are not processed.
- Whole grain pasta
- Sweet potatoes are starchy vegetables containing complex carbohydrates. The best cooking method is baking.

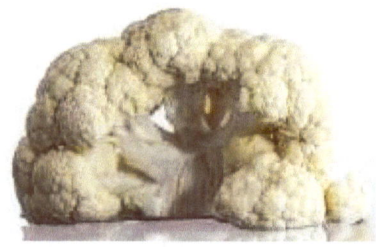

- Beans, peas, and lentils can be added to salads or soups to make a food high in complex carbohydrates, very low in fat and high in fiber and protein.

- Pumpkin— is high in fiber and rich in nutrients, and has a low glycemic index.

The Glycemic Index

The Glycemic Index is a scale that measures a food's impact on raising blood sugars. Insulin trigger foods are typically high on the GI scale. High glycemic foods are those that absorb sugar very quickly into the bloodstream, raising insulin levels immediately and drastically.

Low glycemic index foods are those that contain fiber or that have complex carbohydrates in them so the sugar doesn't digest as fast. You still need to watch calories but, by staying away from high glycemic foods, you will stimulate the pancreatic beta cells much less and less of the sugar will turn into fat.

Low GI foods are recommended for anyone looking to keep Type 2 diabetes at bay and manage their weight.

Carbohydrates are a group of food necessary for survival along with healthy sources of protein and fat. While the USDA dietary guidelines recommended 40-60% of our daily diet come from carbohydrates, many disagree with this formula, and thousands choose to eat a much lower daily carb intake, be it for weight loss, weight maintenance or to prevent or control Type 2 diabetes.

Carbohydrates can be an important part of a well-balanced diet, however studies have shown that they can and do contribute to weight gain in the following ways.

Water Retention

Once the body converts carbs into glucose that is used for fuel, any leftover fuel is then converted into glycogen. Glycogen is stored in the liver and muscles so it can be turned into glucose, as the body needs it. This process results in muscle tissues holding on to extra water that can tip the scale in an unfavorable direction.

Insulin Triggers

When it comes to weight gain, simple sugars are definitely your main culprit. They include any high sugar fruits, and processed foods made from sugar, such as cookies, candy, pies, and pastries, juices and soda. It is estimated that there are about 10 teaspoons of sugar in just one can of sugar-containing soda. Soda is one of the worst drinks because it floods the bloodstream with sugar and secondarily, insulin. Insulin in high quantities attempts to put glucose in the cells for cellular fuel and replenishes the glycogen stores, which is one way of storing sugar.

When there is enough glucose in the cells and enough glycogen has been made, insulin puts the excess sugar into fat cells and turns the glucose into fat. You gain weight and gain fat, especially from eating or drinking foods that contain empty sugar calories that don't really provide you with the minerals and vitamins your body needs.

Good Carbs Versus Bad Carbs

Complex carbohydrates are slow to digest and the metabolism needs time to break these sugars down into simple sugars, primarily glucose, for absorption and for use as fuel.

Complex carbohydrates are considered "good carbs" because they have lots of fiber, vitamins, minerals, and antioxidants and because they do not cause high spikes in blood sugar after eating them.

Starches like whole grains, beans, lentils and whole grain rice or pasta typically fall under the category of "good carbs," and depending on your goals should be included in a well-balanced diet.

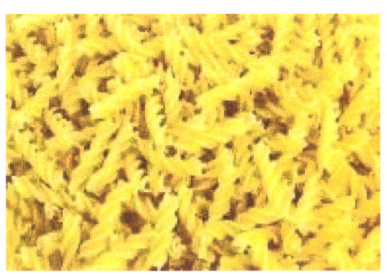

Vegetables are the healthiest carbs and should be incorporated into your diet as much as possible too. This is true whether you want to lose or maintain a healthy weight.

"Bad carbs" are those carbohydrates high on the GI scale that involve simple sugars, which absorb quickly into the bloodstream, allowing insulin to be pumped quickly out of the pancreas in order to lower the blood sugar. Some sugar is used for fuel, other sugar molecules are used to replenish stores of glycogen in the liver, while the leftover sugar goes to make fat. Baked goods, soda, juice, white rice, potatoes, white pasta, and white bread all contribute to weight gain, especially when one overindulges.

Whole grain starches, like brown rice, wild rice, and whole grain bread is a better choice because the fiber is not stripped away from them during processing, as is the case in the white varieties, and the high fiber count helps to counteract the impact of the sugar carbs and keeps you fuller longer.

Some carbohydrates are both good and bad. For example, whole fruits contain the simple sugar fructose, but also contain fiber, which can trap the sugars in the GI tract for a while, so sugar enters the bloodstream more gradually. This is why whole fruit have a lower glycemic index than juice made from the same fruit. Fruits also vary in how many sugar carbs they have with berries having the lowest amount.

The difference between starch and sugar digestion, and thus satiety, can make you eat more food than you need and therefore cause weight gain. Sugars from junk foods digest very fast causing you to feel hungry soon after eating.

Carbs that also contain soluble fiber slow digestion and sugar absorption reducing blood sugar spikes and so vegetables and grains take longer to convert into glucose, which stabilizes your appetite and reduces binge eating.

The Role Of Fiber

Fiber plays a key role in the impact a particular carb content of a food will have on weight gain. Fiber is also the reason that brown whole grains are recommended over processed white grains because the processing strips the grain of fiber, leaving higher impact carbs.

The fiber found in whole fruit is also the reason it is better than juicing that strips away the fiber rich pulp of the fruit making juice higher in sugar impact carbs than eating the whole fruit.

In general, the more fiber a food has, the less impact its carbs will have on blood sugars and the fuller it will keep you.

The formula is simple: when reading food labels subtract the fiber content from the carbohydrate content and that is the actual count of carbs that impact blood sugars and can cause weight gain.

In this case, the actual carb count is 26g – 5g=21g

Foods High In Fiber

- Vegetables, especially green and leafy green varieties
- Berries
- Nuts and seeds
- Dried beans and peas
- Whole grains like bread, whole grain flours, and crackers
- Brown rice and wild rice
- Wheat bran and whole oats
- Quinoa

Nutrition Facts

Serving Size 8 oz (227 g/8 oz)
Servings Per Container About 3

Amount Per Serving

Calories 180   Calories from Fat 60

	% Daily Value*
Total Fat 6g	10 %
Saturated Fat 1g	5 %
Trans Fat 0g	
Cholesterol 5mg	2 %
Sodium 75mg	3 %
Total Carbohydrate 26g	9 %
Dietary Fiber 5g	19 %
Sugars 11g	
Protein 8g	

Vitamin A 60%	•	Vitamin C 70%
Calcium 8%	•	Iron 10%

* Percent Daily Values are based on a 2,000 calorie diet. Your daily values may be higher or lower depending on your calorie needs.

	Calories	2,000	2,500
Total Fat	Less than	65g	80g
Sat Fat	Less than	20g	25g
Cholesterol	Less than	300mg	300mg
Sodium	Less than	2,400mg	2,400mg
Total Carbohydrate		300g	375g
Dietary Fiber		25g	30g

Calories per gram:
Fat 9 • Carbohydrate 4 • Protein 4

When considering a low carb diet for weight loss, most plans place a great emphasis on vegetables as main carb sources, with whole grains coming in second, if at all since they still have more impact on blood glucose than vegetable carbs, and so portion size is important.

The other benefit of fiber is that it keeps you full longer, so over the course of a day you eat less, another benefit for weight management. In addition, eating a diet low in carbs and high in fiber helps to alleviate those out of control cravings for unhealthy junk food – another plus when trying to manage weight.

Low Carb Weight Loss

Low carb diets are often used for weight loss, and they have experienced a high level of popularity in recent years ... so much so that those looking to maintain a healthy weight and keep their blood sugar healthy to prevent diabetes have also adopted this type of eating style.

Typically in a low carb diet, the menu significantly reduces complex carbs and completely eliminates simple carbs. Most of the carbs in a low carb diet come from high fiber, low carb vegetables. Allowances differ from one diet to the next, such as the case with Atkins that prescribes an induction phase that eliminates all grains, and only allows vegetables as carb sources.

Typical Menu

- In general, low carb diets include meat, poultry, fish and seafood protein, eggs, and non-starchy vegetables.

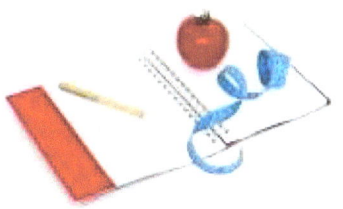

- Generally, grains, nuts, and beans are limited and simple sugars are eliminated.

Carb Allowance

Some diets initially restrict and then gradually increase the number of allowed carbs, such as Atkins in the Induction Phase that allows only 20 net carbs in the first two weeks. Conversely, other plans maintain the same daily limit of carbs from the beginning.

While the Dietary Guidelines for Americans recommends that 45% to 65% of an adult diet come from carbs, which equals to 225 to 325 grams of carbs daily based on a 2,000 calorie diet, a low carb diet (depending on the particular plan) set limits that range from only 20 to 130 grams of carbs allowed daily. The very low carb plans will restrict carbs to 60 grams or less per day.

Low carb diets are generally considered high fat diets, with approximately 40% to 75% of calories acquired from fats, 20% from protein, and about 5% from carbohydrates.

Do low carb diets result in weight loss? Yes, they do and there is solid science behind them. However many of them are so restrictive that they are non-sustainable over a long period of time. Once off of the diet, many people gain the weight they lost right back. A better plan is to eat healthy with the right balance of complex carbs, protein and unsaturated fats – 50%, 30% and 20% respectively is a good place to start and adjust from there as your body dictates.

Lipolysis and Ketosis

Lipolysis occurs when the body begins to burn fat stores for energy instead of carbohydrates that are obtained from meals. The by-products of this fat burning process are ketones and ketosis is the secondary process of lipolysis.

By depriving the body of carbohydrates, which are converted to glucose and typically used as fuel, it is forced to use its fat stores instead, literally melting it off the body in a state referred to as ketosis.

According to Dr. Atkins, creator of the Atkins Diet...

"If you're not in ketosis, you're in "glucosis."

Lipolysis is the most efficient biochemical path to weight loss and the scientifically proven alternative to using glucose for energy.

The only exception to the body not needing glucose for fuel is ketones.

Lipolysis and the secondary process of ketosis provides adequate fuel for cells, the brain and other organs (just as glucose from carbs does) BUT, it allows the body to burn stored fat for energy resulting in weight loss and healthy weight management.

Ketone production occurs when insulin in the bloodstream is low. The lower the insulin level, the higher the ketone production and vice versa. This process of optimal ketosis can only occur while following a low carb diet, sometimes referred to as a ketogenic diet or ket diet.

What The Science Shows

Ketogenic or low carb diets do result in weight loss. One study conducted in 2008 and published in the American Journal of Clinical Nutrition documented a 12 pound weight loss in only 4 weeks in obese men who followed such an eating plan. The subjects noted that they had less hunger while eating fewer calories.

A National Center For Complementary and Integrative Health funded study at Stanford University (Christopher Gardner, et al) followed 311 pre-menopausal women, all of whom were overweight or obese. Each woman was randomly assigned one of four diets, which included, the Atkins diet, the Zone diet, the LEARN diet and the Ornish diet. Atkins was the lowest carb diet, the Zone diet is also a low carb diet, but higher in carbs than Atkins and the other two were normal carb, but low fat diets.

The results showed that the Atkins group of women lost the most weight with an average of 10 pounds over 12 months. The Atkins group also showed better metabolic effects.

Another study from Duke University Medical Center followed 120 obese subjects who did the Atkins diet and lost an average of 31 pounds after six months, while those who followed the American Heart Association's low-fat plan lost only 20 pounds.

Atkins diet statistics published in 2003 in the distinguished *New England Journal of Medicine* stated that people on the Atkins diet lost twice as much weight during a six-month period as people who followed a low-fat diet.

The Mayo Clinic confirms that a ketogenic diet could have favorable effects on cardiovascular disease, diabetes, and metabolic syndrome. Furthermore, a low carb diet can improve levels of bad LDL cholesterol better than moderate-carbohydrate diets.

However, are any of the low carb diets sustainable over a long period of time? Most are not. Losing weight slow by eating healthy is still the best way to lose weight and keep it off.

Benefits of Low Carb Diets

With the staggering rise in Type 2 diabetes, as reported by the American Diabetes Association, current numbers are 29.1 million Americans, or 9.3% of the population diagnosed; that doesn't include the thousands that are prediabetic or the diabetics not yet diagnosed. Because of these numbers, more and more attention is being paid to low carb, higher protein diets.

In truth, all people need carbohydrates, protein, and fat to some degree but, in a low carb diet, the emphasis is on healthy fats and lean meats, and other forms of protein instead of carbohydrates.

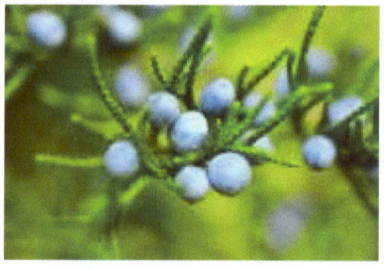

A low carb diet focuses on protein and healthy fats as a source of nutrition, eliminating simple carbohydrates and having almost all carbohydrates in the complex form, so there are no blood sugar spikes that can lead to fat deposition and Type 2 diabetes.

Very low carb diets, such as the South Beach and Atkins have helped people lose weight because they provide minimal increases in blood sugar and insulin so that less of the food goes to fat. Because low carb eating creates a state of ketosis within the body, it burns stored fat for energy instead of carbohydrates from food.

Low carb diets incorporate complex carbohydrates such as whole grains, oats, green vegetables, pumpkin, corn, and beans—all of which digest slowly and contain a great deal of plant fiber that doesn't get digested; the undigested fiber helps bowel movements come more easily and regularly. Sugars found in these complex carbohydrates are long chain sugars that need to be broken down in the digestive tract before the simple sugars can be absorbed by the duodenum and small intestines. This gradual process eliminates wide fluctuations in sugar and insulin.

Prevent Chronic Disease

We know eating a low carb and healthy carb diet is the best way to prevent Type 2 diabetes. Low-carb diets may also play a key role in preventing and improving serious health conditions, including metabolic syndrome, high blood pressure, and cardiovascular disease.

Of course, any diet that results in weight loss will reduce risk for and may prevent heart disease and diabetes. Evidence exists that low-carb diets may also lower bad LDL cholesterol and triglyceride values a little more than diets with moderate carb counts. However, the American College of Cardiology and The American Heart Association believe that not enough evidence exists to suggest that low-carbohydrate diets have heart health benefits.

Ketosis And Type 2 Diabetes

Nutritionists often recommend a ketogenic diet for patients who have Type 2 diabetes where the body is unable to properly use the insulin it makes to process glucose in the bloodstream.

A ketogenic diet reduces carbohydrate intake that can stabilize blood sugar levels. However, care should be taken and those with diabetes should only follow a keto diet under the supervision of a physician as a serious life-threatening condition called ketoacidosis can occur if ketone levels get too high.

Weight Loss

Many people have had success in losing weight on a low carb diet. When insulin levels are kept low, this promotes the breakdown of fat into fuel instead of the other way around. Protein and healthy fats do not stimulate insulin so fatty deposition does not happen as readily.

Low carb diets tend to eliminate highly processed, fat, and sugar-containing foods, which are high in calories. The total calorie count is what really matters in weight loss and foods high in meat protein, vegetable protein, and healthy plant fats keep you feeling sated longer so you don't feel the need to overeat.

A typical low carb diet consists of lean meats, eggs, dairy, fresh whole fruits and vegetables. The whole fruits and vegetables contain a lot of fiber, which also lends itself to keeping you feeling fuller for longer periods. You tend 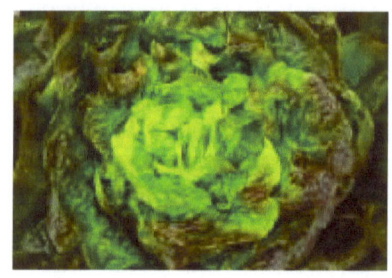 to eat less because you are full quicker and a slow and gradual weight loss pattern emerges.

Low carb diets also eliminate the use of sugar-containing sodas that contain large amounts of simple sugars and that raise insulin levels very quickly. Even though there is no fat in these carbonated sodas, the high sugar content cannot possibly be used up by the cells nor can it be stored safely in the liver as glycogen.

The body wants to keep the blood sugars as normal as possible so the excess glucose you taken in with sugar-containing sodas just goes to build up fat in your system. High protein and high essential fatty acid diets just don't have this problem. Other health benefits of a low carb diet include:

- Reduction in hunger

- Enhanced mental functioning

- Lower risk for certain kinds of cancer

- A loss of body fat, most predominantly from around the abdomen

- Increased level of "good" cholesterol (HDL)

- A healthy blood pressure level

(NOTE – There is no guarantee that a low carb diet will deliver any of the health benefits just discussed. However, those wonderful health advantages listed above, and others, have been experienced by a majority of people that cut back on their carbohydrate intake in a safe and sensible manner.)

Carbs and Blood Sugar

Many people don't realize Type 2 diabetics can have as many spikes in blood sugar as are seen in Type 1. In Type 2, the problem isn't too much or too little insulin but a chronic insulin resistance that reveals itself in spikes of blood sugar when the Type 2 diabetic eats too many simple carbohydrates.

Simple carbohydrates are the same thing as simple sugars. They include sugars like glucose, galactose, fructose, and sucrose. Of these, only sucrose is actually two simple sugars linked together but, as the molecule is still small, it can be absorbed by the gastrointestinal tract just like glucose. All sugars eventually end up as glucose, which is used by fuel for the cells.

In the case of Type 2 diabetics, when glucose floods the system after a high sugar meal, insulin levels rise but the insulin is unable to put the sugar into the cells for cellular fuel and the blood sugar spikes.

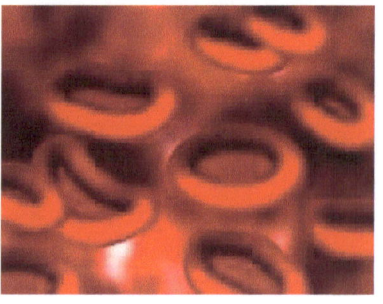

Some of the sugar is used to replenish glycogen stores in the liver but most ends up turning to fat. This is why many Type 2 diabetics have a lot of fat on their body because the insulin has no place to put the spikes in glucose.

Type 2 diabetics need to monitor their intake of simple sugars in such a way as to avoid the intake of simple sugars as much as possible. Simple sugars are found in any product to which table sugar is added. For example, drinking one can of sugared soda is the equivalent of eating up to ten teaspoons of sugar. All of this sugar floods the blood system at once, overloading the pancreas, and spiking sugars. The same is true when Type 2 diabetics eat too much candy, cakes, cookies, pies, and pastries that are made with a lot of sugar.

Many ice creams contain a great deal of sugar as well. All of these foods have a high glycemic index, meaning that they flood the bloodstream with sugar very quickly, forcing a sudden increase in ineffectively working insulin. The spike goes down as the insulin turns the extra glucose to fat.

In the meantime, high blood sugar and Type 2 diabetes can cause end-organ damage, such as kidney disease, peripheral vascular disease, heart disease, diabetic neuropathy, and diabetic retinopathy and take years off the diabetic's life.

Diabetics who do not exercise will experience glucose spikes as well. Exercise helps put sugar into cells so that sedentary diabetics will not be able to use all the sugar they take in. This is especially true for those who eat mostly simple sugars.

Alternatives To Simple Sugars

Diabetics do not have to avoid carbohydrates altogether. In fact, the American Diabetes Association recommends that diabetics eat complex carbohydrates, which in general do not cause great fluctuations in blood sugar.

Remember that complex carbohydrates are long chain sugars that can't absorb in the body until they are broken up into smaller pieces in the gastrointestinal tract. This takes time and the blood sugar generally rises much more slowly.

If fiber is added to the mix, more delay is granted to the gastrointestinal tract and there is even less of a glucose spike because fiber holds onto sugars, letting them go gradually as the food passes through the gastrointestinal tract.

Complex carbohydrates in foods such as brown rice, whole-wheat pasta, whole wheat bread products, beans, quinoa, and many non-starchy vegetables work well; avoid the juice of fruits and stick to the fruit itself.

The whole fruit contains fiber, which is what keeps the simple sugar in the gut longer than the juice, which drastically increases the glucose spike noted after drinking it.

If a majority of your diet is carbohydrate-rich foods, you are going to need to replace them with something. The following swaps move you from carb-heavy foods to low carb alternatives.

1 - Instead of sugar, use …

Stevia, coconut palm sugar, raw honey or molasses.

2 – Instead of white flour, use …

Almond flour.

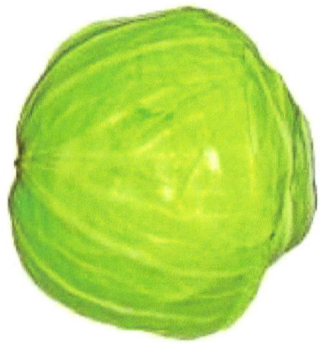

3 - Instead of taco shells, use ...

Leafy greens like kale, cabbage, lettuce and collard leaves.

4 - Instead of hamburger buns, use ...

Portabello mushroom caps.

5 - Instead of sliced bread, use ...

Slices of eggplant.

6 - Instead of french fries, use ...

Turnips, butternut squash or carrots.

7 - Instead of lasagna, use ...

Eggplant or zucchini.

8 - Instead of mashed potatoes or macaroni and cheese, use ...

Cauliflower.

9 - Instead of pancakes, use ...

Oatmeal cakes.

10 - Instead of pizza crust, use ...

Cauliflower or mushrooms.

11 - Instead of pasta, use ...

Shirataki noodles or butternut squash noodles.

How to Start a Low Carb Diet

Before starting a low carb diet, you have to ask yourself *"How many carbohydrates should I be eating?"* That seems like a rather basic question that probably has a simple answer. The opposite is actually true. The number of carbohydrates you eat is important, but as you learned, the kinds of carbohydrates you eat dictate your health as well.

Nutritionists, doctors and other health experts in the United Kingdom, the US and most other modern countries agree on your basic daily carbohydrate quantity. They should comprise somewhere between 45% and 65% of your total calorie count each day. This means you must first calculate how many calories you should be consuming on a daily basis.

How Many Calories Do You Really Need?

Each human being is vastly different metabolically. Two people the same size, weight, age and gender could have totally different metabolisms. So **use the following formula for determining your daily calorie intake simply as a guide.** It should be used as a jumping off point, with you listening to your body and tweaking accordingly.

First you will need to calculate your basal metabolic rate (BMR). You do this using the Harris Benedict principle.

- **For Women -** Multiply your weight (in pounds) by 4.3. Add 655 to that number. Multiply your height (in inches) by 4.7. Add that number to your previous total. Multiply your age (in years) by 4.7, and subtract that number from your total.

Here is the BMR formula made simple. *655 + (4.3 x weight in pounds) + (4.7 x height in inches) - (4.7 x age in years)*

- **For Men -** *66 + (6.3 x weight in pounds) + (12.9 x height in inches) - (6.8 x age in years)*

Now you need to factor in your activity level.

- If you are sedentary (very little to no exercise), multiply your BMR by 1.2.

- If you are lightly active (some exercise), multiply your BMR by 1.3.

- If you are moderately active (you exercise most days of the week), multiply your BMR by 1.4.

- If you are very active (you enjoy intense exercise for prolonged periods of time 5 to 7 days a week), multiply your BMR by 1.5 or 1.6.

The result of all that math is the number of calories you need to eat each day to maintain your current weight. If your head is hurting just looking at those formulas, try this instead. Type *"calorie calculator"* into your favorite search engine, fill in the blanks, and you will instantly see how many daily calories you need to consume.

Let's say you discover you need to eat 1,500 calories each day to stay at your current weight. To lose weight, you'll have to eat fewer. As you learned earlier, between 45% and 65% of that calorie count should come from carbohydrates. That means 675 to 975 of your daily calories should be carbohydrates.

Remember, find your daily recommended calorie intake first. Then figure between 45% and 65% of that number. This is the number of daily carbohydrate calories you should be eating. Just make sure that the vast majority of your carbohydrates are complex, instead of simple carbs.

Now that we know how many carbs we should be eating , let's move on to low carb diets. Not all commercial low carb diets are the same, as some are stricter than others are in the foods they allow and the total daily carb intake.

Commercial Low Carb Diets

- Atkins Nutritional Program (lowest carb intake with 4 phases that increase carb intake gradually)
- The Ketogenic Diet (high-fat, adequate-protein, low-carbohydrate)
- Glycemic Index Diet (focuses on eating low GI foods)
- The South Beach Diet (focuses on healthy carbs)
- The Zone Diet (allows 40% carbs)
- Nutrisystem Diet (based on low glycemic index with a balance of protein, carbs and fats)
- Dukan Diet (low carb long term plan)
- ITG Diet (3-step diet that limits carbs and targets a healthy balanced diet for long term weight maintenance)

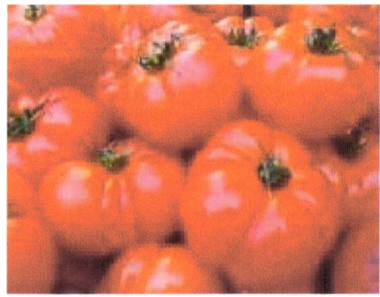

You can start a low carb diet today simply be ridding your kitchen of highly processed foods that contain a high sugar content. Eat a wide variety of non-starchy vegetables, along with non-fried steak, chicken, seafood, fish, and eggs. Drink water, and plain tea instead of sugar-containing sodas.

Low Carb Versus Low Fat Diets

You can find information all over the web and in books about various diets and their claims. There are low carb diets, low fat diets, and low calorie diets. It can be difficult to know exactly which diet is best for you with all this information around. Certainly, low carb and low fat eating plans are two of the most popular, and have been compared in studies many times over. Of course, there are pros and cons to both.

Low Carb Diet

There are many proprietary low carb diets, which are based on the idea that carbohydrates trigger insulin and cause insulin/glucose spikes. With spikes in glucose and insulin, much of the glucose in the carbohydrate diet goes to make fat. With a low carb diet, the glucose levels fluctuate less and insulin/fat production is minimized.

In low carb diets, the emphasis is placed on eating lean meats, alternative sources of protein, healthy fats and a limited amount of complex carbohydrates. Simple carbohydrates like glucose, fructose, galactose, and sucrose (table sugar) are eliminated from the diet, which eliminates many foods that are high in calories.

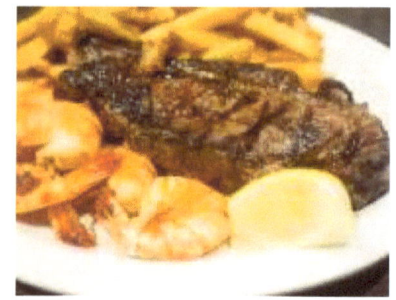

Sugar-containing sodas, donuts, cake and all foods containing table sugar are completely out of the picture in a low carb diet, which means people drink more water and more unsweetened beverages, which are naturally low in calories (and better for you).

These diets allow much more fat than low fat diets. Some of the fat comes from animal protein sources and ideally, a lot of the fat comes from unsaturated plant sources like olive oil, cottonseed oil, and other vegetable oils. Oils that are high in polyunsaturated fats are less demanding on the arteries, producing less arterial plaques than, say, saturated fats that come from meat sources.

Still, the content of low carb diets is much fattier than low fat or high carb diets and, while these types of food taste good, some would argue that too much fat brings on too many calories to the diet. Fat is 9 calories per gram while protein and carbohydrates are only 4 calories per gram. This means that even a little bit of fat has twice the calories than either protein or carbohydrates. However, the proponents of low carb eating argue that since the body is burning stored fat for fuel instead of carbs from food, weight loss is inevitable.

Weight loss in a low carb diet tends to be slower than with a low fat diet because the calorie counts in low carb diets are still somewhat elevated from a strictly low calorie diet. On the other hand, protein helps keep a person fuller for a longer period of time so there is a tendency to eat less.

It is also a fact that once one reaches a state of ketosis, fat loss can be quite rapid and people who follow these diets report having an abundance of energy, a significant reduction in out of control cravings (stable blood sugars) and they feel full and satisfied with less food.

Low Fat Diet

Low fat diets, on the other hand, contain a great deal of plant

carbohydrates. Plant foods like fruits and vegetables contain very little fat and yet because of the fiber, can fill you up. You can read the label on just about anything and count fat grams, limiting fat content per day to 10-20 fat grams.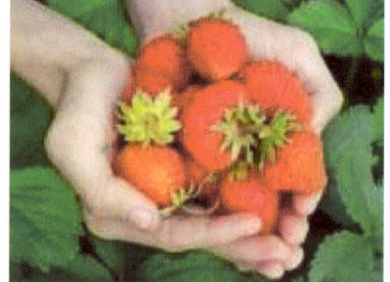

You'll find that many fatty meats and fried food is out of the picture in a low fat diet and weight loss tends to be more rapid.

The food may be less appetizing and you don't get the satisfaction of eating foods containing fat, but this type of diet is tolerable for those who enjoy eating lots of fruits, vegetables, fish, and de-skinned poultry.

Low fat diets tend to be harder to maintain over the long haul. There is fat in just about any type of meat and in things like beans and nuts, so you have to eliminate or greatly reduce these from your diet in order to keep the fat grams down.

Your skin tends to dry out when on low fat diets and, while you may lose weight, you are also missing out on plant-based oils, which contain omega 3 and omega 6 fatty acids. You need those fatty acids for cellular metabolism and to keep the cell membranes healthy so a low fat diet typically should be supplemented with vitamins. And don't forget that to process and absorb the fat-soluble vitamins, A, K, E,D, you need a certain amount of fat in your diet.

What Diet Is Better?

While several studies have proven low carb diets to yield more weight loss in subjects than low fat varieties, in the end, the best diet is the one that you can stick with for life. When paired with exercise and a reduction of unhealthy habits, it is called healthy living and something you can sustain forever.

In truth, either the low carb or the low fat diet can be detrimental to an individual because certain foods are eliminated, and so it may be hard to stick with.

The best diet for you is one that contains foods you learn to like that are low in calories and dense in nutrients.

You need fats, protein and some complex carbohydrates in any diet so the trick is deciding which your prefer, and what works better for you in maintaining satiety, high levels of energy and weight loss.

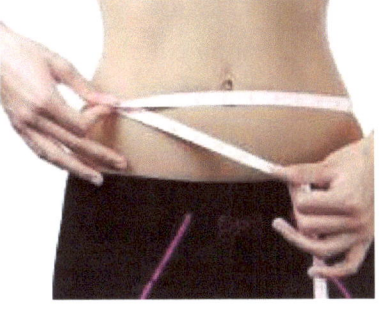

Bottom Line

Learning about carbohydrates and how they impact the body is important to ensure you enjoy good health and gain all the benefits of a healthy body weight.

Carbohydrates are important nutrients; however, choosing healthy carbs is critical in preventing obesity, Type 2 diabetes and many of the conditions associated with these. Consider for a moment how much sugar you eat every day, and likely like millions of others, you eat too much.

Low carb eating is used by millions of people around the world, and it maybe something that can be of benefit to you. Don't forget to ask your doctor first!

Carbohydrates are not inherently evil. They are not good or bad either. When you eat too many of the wrong types of carbohydrates however, health problems can appear. That is why it is important to eat lots of complex carbohydrates, and less simple carbs. I've included this carbs checklist that is a quick way to tell you everything you need to know about carbohydrates, which ones to avoid and eat more of, and how to determine how many carbohydrates you should eat every day.

Here is a handy checklist you can use as a quick reference:

☐ Carbohydrates are most people's main source of energy.

☐ Healthy fats are a smart replacement for carbohydrates as a source of energy.

☐ Every cell in your body, and all body tissue, needs carbohydrates to work properly.

☐ However, when you eat too many carbohydrates, your body stores excess blood sugar as fat.

☐ Carbohydrates are 1 of 3 macronutrients your body needs. The other 2 are protein and fat.

☐ There are 3 kinds of carbohydrates – sugars, fibers and starches.

☐ Those 3 types of carbs are either simple carbohydrates or complex carbohydrates.

☐ Simple carbs are sugars. They have a simple chemical construction, so they are processed very rapidly. This leads to greater storage of fat.

☐ Complex carbs are starches. They are complex in makeup, so it takes longer for your body to process them. This leads to less storage of fat.

☐ Simple carbs have little to no nutritional value, and lead to overweight and obesity when eaten in abundance.

☐ Complex carbs are rich in nutrients and minerals, and lead to a healthy body weight regulation when eaten in abundance.

A low carb eating approach offers the following health benefits...

✓ Reduction in hunger
✓ Enhanced mental functioning

- ✓ Lower risk of contracting heart disease
- ✓ Lower risk for certain kinds of cancer
- ✓ A loss of body fat, most predominantly from around the abdomen
- ✓ Increased level of "good" cholesterol (HDL)
- ✓ A healthy blood pressure level

Take care and stay well!

Quick Low Carb Recipe Suggestions

Broccoli Soup With Carrots Recipe

This is a recipe for broccoli soup with carrots, which has flavor from the onions and garlic in it. This is a very simple recipe and very tasty too. You can choose to add more vegetables of your choice.

What You'll Need:

- ✓ ¼ cup onion, chopped
- ✓ 2 garlic cloves, chopped
- ✓ ½ cup carrots
- ✓ 1 cup broccoli florets
- ✓ 1 tbsp. oil
- ✓ 3 cups of water
- ✓ Salt, pepper and lemon juice as per taste

Method:

1. Heat oil in pan, then add the garlic and sauté for 2 minutes.
2. Add onion and sauté for 5 minutes.
3. Add carrots and salt, and sauté for 5 minutes.
4. Add broccoli and sauté for 5 minutes.
5. Add water and let it boil.
6. Once it has boiled, let it simmer for 10 minutes on low heat.
7. Add pepper and lemon juice.
8. Serve hot.

Chicken Stir-Fry Recipe

An easy and fast recipe for weekday dinners need not be boring. Try this chicken stir-fry and get dinner done in less than 30 minutes including prep!

What You'll Need:

- ✓ ½ pound chicken breast, sliced thinly.
- ✓ 1 to 1 1/2 cup baby corn sliced diagonally
- ✓ 1 medium sized red bell pepper cut into strips
- ✓ 1 small bundle of green onion cut into two inch long pieces (about ½ cup or a bit more)
- ✓ 1 to 1 ½ cup sugar snap peas (also goes by chicharo or snow peas)
- ✓ 1 tablespoon soybean oil or any light cooking oil
- ✓ 2 tablespoons coconut aminos

Let's Make Some Awesome Chicken Stir-Fry!

1. Cut up and wash everything in advance. This recipe goes pretty fast in the cooking department so make sure all veggies are ready to go.
2. Heat your wok or heavy bottom frying pan over medium to high heat and brown the sliced chicken breast on all sides.
3. Add the ginger.
4. Sauté until the ginger's flavor has infused with the chicken.
5. Add the baby corn and the white and thick parts of the green onion then sauté for about a minute.

Make sure to keep everything moving on the pan or wok so that it won't burn.

6. Add the coconut aminos.
7. And stir, stir, stir!
8. In the last minute, add the sugar snap peas, red bell pepper, and the green stalks of the green onion. Don't cook for longer than a minute at this point.
9. Serve hot. Make it pretty with some optional sesame seeds and a drizzle of sesame oil.

This recipe makes 2 servings.

Grilled Garlic Broccoli Recipe

This is a very simple and tasty recipe. It is nice way to enjoy broccoli with the pure flavor of garlic.

Ingredients:

- ✓ 1 cup broccoli florets
- ✓ 6-8 garlic cloves
- ✓ 2 tbsp. olive oil
- ✓ Salt and pepper to taste

Method:

1. Marinate broccoli florets for 30 minutes with olive oil and salt, so that they become tender.

2. Pre-heat the oven at 175 C (350 F) for 5 minutes.

3. In a baking tray, place the broccoli florets and garlic cloves.

4. Place the tray in the oven at 175 C (350 F) for 10 minutes.

5. Toss the broccoli and bake for further 10-15 minutes or until broccoli is cooked and crispy.

6. Serve warm.

Tips:

1. You may add more veggies like carrots, zucchini etc.

2. Keep a watch on the broccoli while it's being cooked to ensure it does not get burned.

Serves: 2
Preparation time: 30 minutes

Grilled Shrimp Salad Recipe

Fancy a fresh tasting, tangy and sweet light seafood salad? Try this Asian grilled shrimp salad for brunch or even a picnic. The combination of the smoky grilled flavor from the grilled shrimp, the slightly sweet and salty shrimp taste, plus the tart and spicy dressing makes for a feast your senses will surely love.

What You Will Need:

- ✓ 1 small head of lettuce, leaves separated (romaine or ice berg lettuce)
- ✓ 1 small red onion, sliced thinly
- ✓ 1 cup of medium sized shrimps, deveined, cleaned and without shell
- ✓ 1 teaspoon sesame seeds
- ✓ 1-3 teaspoons of wasabi paste, adjust according to taste
- ✓ 3 tablespoons red wine vinegar
- ✓ 1 tablespoon mayonnaise
- ✓ 1 tablespoon sesame oil
- ✓ 1 tablespoon vegetable oil
- ✓ 3 cloves of garlic, finely chopped

Time for Some Awesome Shrimp Salad!

1. Gather all the needed ingredients together.
2. Coat the shrimps with the vegetable oil, garlic, and half the sesame oil.
3. Grill on a pan or stove top grill.
4. For the dressing, combine the wasabi paste, mayonnaise and red wine vinegar.
5. To assemble the salad, lay down the lettuce leaves, sprinkle the red onions over it and add the cooked shrimp. Drizzle the dressing over the salad and sprinkle the sesame seeds. Don't forget to drizzle half of the sesame oil to give it an extra layer of flavor!
6. Serves two persons. Enjoy!

Oven Roasted Beef-Wrapped Asparagus Recipe

For an easy and fast dinner appetizer with a mix of eastern and western flavors, try this roasted beef wrapped asparagus which comes together in less than an hour. With this recipe, there is no excuse for not impressing guests at your dinner table even if it is an after-work-hours gathering.

What You'll Need:

- ✓ ½ lb Beef sliced thinly or sukiyaki style
- ✓ 1 bundle asparagus spears
- ✓ ½ teaspoon freshly cracked blacked pepper
- ✓ ½ teaspoon red chili flakes
- ✓ 1 teaspoon sesame seeds
- ✓ 1 tablespoon sesame oil
- ✓ 1 tablespoon vegetable oil
- ✓ 1 tablespoon soy sauce
- ✓ 1 small piece of ginger (makes about 1 teaspoon of grated ginger)
- ✓ 2 cloves of garlic

Let's Wrap Em Asparagus!

1. Make sure you got all the ingredients that you need ready.
2. In a bowl, grate the ginger and garlic.
3. Add in the beef, soy sauce, chili flakes, freshly cracked black pepper, vegetable oil, and sesame seeds.
4. Mix together and let stand for 15 minutes while you clean and cut up the asparagus stalks.

5. Wrap each asparagus stalk with a piece of beef while you preheat the oven at 200C. You may also use the grill or broiler.
6. Here they are all wrapped up!
7. Arrange on a baking tray at least an inch apart if using the oven. They can be grilled on the griller too especially if you have an outdoor party or gathering. Bake for 15 minutes or until the asparagus are tender but not soggy and the beef is cooked through.
8. Serve up as is or with some sriracha for an added kick! Don't forget to drizzle in some sesame oil just before serving.
9. Enjoy this eastern inspired beef-wrapped asparagus!

Radish With Sesame Seed Salad Recipe

Radish with Sesame Paste Salad is something I grew up eating. It and can be eaten with bread or rice. It takes just 10 minutes to make it but the taste is amazing. So let's get started!

Ingredients:

- ✓ Radish
- ✓ Onion - 1
- ✓ Green Chilies - 3
- ✓ Sesame Seed Paste – 2 tbsps.
- ✓ Coriander Leaves
- ✓ Lemon – Half
- ✓ Salt to Taste

Preparation:

1. Get all your ingredients ready.

2. Wash the radish under running water, then using a potato peeler, peel the cover of the radish.

3. Once done, cut the entire radish and the stem into 2 cms long thin pieces.

4. Soak the radish in a salt water to reduce the gas in it. Leave it for at least 10 minutes.

5. Also cut the onion and chilies into thin long pieces, then cut the coriander into small pieces.

6. Then mix all the ingredients together and then add 2 tbsp. of sesame seed paste.

7. Mix it properly and then add the salt to taste.

8. For the final touch, squeeze half a lemon into the salad.

9. That's all. It's best to let this salad sit in the fridge for 10 minutes so the flavors can mix well. Enjoy! Serve at room temperature. Garnish with fresh coriander. Serve hot with mixed vegetables.

Spicy Poached Chicken Recipe

This Chinese-fusion dish is usually served at formal functions and gatherings but you don't need any special event to make this right at your kitchen! All you need is some spices, half an hour of your time, and voila! You have spicy poached chicken!

What You'll Need:

- ✓ 1 to 2 pounds chicken pieces (with the bones in)
- ✓ 1 small stalk of lemongrass
- ✓ Peel of half an orange
- ✓ 1 stalk celery
- ✓ 1 tablespoon whole peppercorns
- ✓ 1 teaspoon caraway seeds
- ✓ 1 ounce piece fresh ginger root
- ✓ 1 red Thai chili
- ✓ 2 green finger chilies
- ✓ 2 pieces star anise
- ✓ Half a red onion
- ✓ 1 teaspoon salt
- ✓ Some water
- ✓ Half a cup light flavored oil (such as palm oil or vegetable oil)

Let's Cook Up Some Spicy Poached Chicken!

1. Begin by placing cleaned chicken pieces in a pot or pan with enough water to cover the chicken. Add in the lemongrass, orange peel, celery, and salt. Bring to a simmer and cook covered for another 15 to 20 minutes.
2. Once done, the chicken can be eaten as is but this won't be spicy poached chicken without the spicy part!

3. For the spicy 'sauce' gather the peppercorns, onion, chilies, star anise, oil, ginger, and caraway seeds. Slice the ginger, onions, and chili.
4. In a small pan over medium heat, place all the spices and the oil. Slowly heat up to infuse the oil with the spices.
5. After about 5 minutes of the spices steeping in the oil, pour the 'sauce' over the drained chicken pieces.
6. You can strain the oil but the traditional way of serving this dish is with all the spices left in the oil, that way, people would know what's in it.
7. This dish is best enjoyed with some steamed rice or some soy sauce fried rice.
8. Don't forget to use the oil as a dipping sauce, you'll be in for a tasty surprise!

Other Senior Health and Fitness Books by This Author

If you would like to read more about Senior Health and Fitness, here is a list of the titles, CreateSpace links and descriptions:

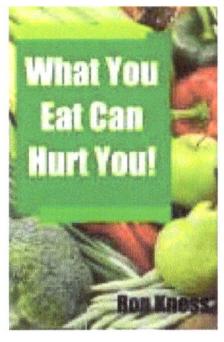

What You Eat Can Hurt You

https://www.createspace.com/4963196

Do you know that certain foods increase your risk for inflammation, disease and illness? It's true! And certain foods can help cure and heal you if you do get sick. Knowing which foods to eat and which ones to avoid empowers you to manage your own health.

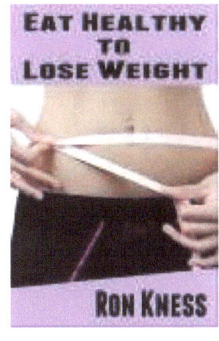

Eat Healthy to Lose Weight

https://www.createspace.com/4962939

As you read through our book, we show you which foods you should and should not be eating to reach your weight loss goal, along with discussing how to maintain your weight loss and stay within a few pounds of your goal weight. Banish the weight you keep gaining back each time by learning how to live a healthy lifestyle.

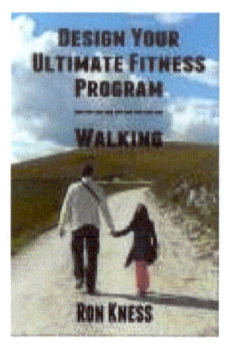

Design Your Ultimate Fitness Program - Walking

https://www.createspace.com/5252272

In my book Design Your Ultimate Fitness Program – Walking, we discuss the considerations that need to be made when designing a custom walking program, along with:
• Equipment needed
• Wearable technology you can use to track your walking
• And how to make walking more challenging

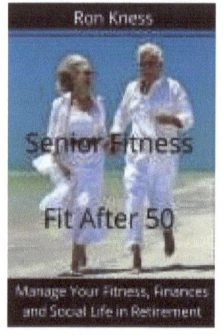

Senior Fitness – Fit After 50: Learn How to Manage Your Fitness, Finances and Social Life in Retirement

https://www.createspace.com/5474751

Inside you will discover answers to your most pressing questions:
• What do I need to know about downsizing my home?
• What are the best tips for staying healthy as you approach your 50's?
• When should I start planning for retirement?

• I am worried about being lonely once I retire, do others feel the same?

• Is it worthwhile to carry two homes during retirement?

And more…

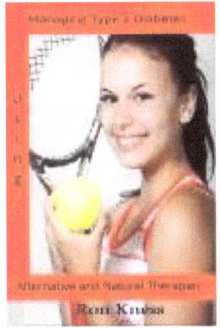 [Managing Type 2 Diabetes Using Alternative And Natural Therapies](https://www.createspace.com/5401244)

https://www.createspace.com/5401244

While Type 2 diabetes can be managed medically, there are many alternative natural and holistic methods of therapy and treatment that can further enhance quality of life and minimize the effects of this disease. In this book, I discuss 12 different types, including yoga, reflexology and acupuncture to name just three.

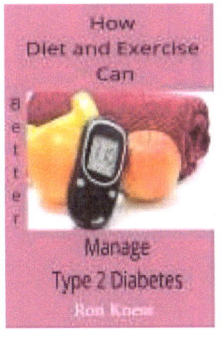 [How Diet and Exercise Can Better Manage Type 2 Diabetes](https://www.createspace.com/5404845)

https://www.createspace.com/5404845

Of the different types of diabetes, only Type 2 can be reversed. In my book How Diet and Exercise Can Better Manage Type 2 Diabetes, we reveal the three things you can do to best manage your disease, including:

• Diet

• Exercise

• Weight management

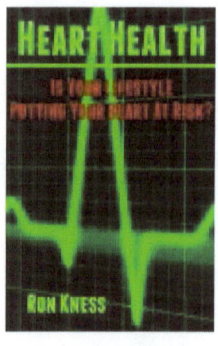

[Heart Health: Is Your Lifestyle Putting Your Heart at Risk?](https://www.createspace.com/5464020)

https://www.createspace.com/5464020

In my ebook Is Your Lifestyle Putting Your Heart At Risk? we discuss the six greatest risks to your heart and the lifestyle changes you can make to mitigate them.

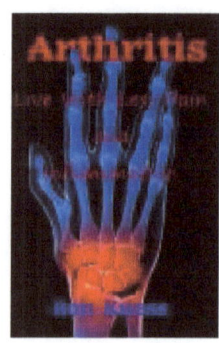

[Arthritis – Live Wth Less Pain and Inflammation: Tips and Techniques You Can Use to Lessen the Pain and Inflammation](https://www.createspace.com/5457441)

https://www.createspace.com/5457441

Discover Simple Tips & Information That Will Help Reduce The Painful Symptoms Of Arthritis!

You learn things like:
• Simple and effective information that will help you manage the pain and inflammation that comes along with arthritis, so that you can live an active, full life without debilitating pain.
• The different types of arthritis, their symptoms and how to alleviate their painful side effects.
• The pros and cons of over-the-counter arthritis medications, plus simple tips that will help you know how to choose the right supplements.

• Free, yet effective ways to get relief from arthritis pain and inflammation, so you don't have to suffer anymore.

the effects arthritis can have significant impact on your physical and mental well-being, but this books shows you how to overcome its painful symptoms and live life relatively pain free.

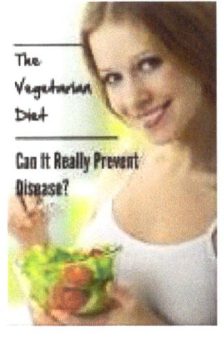

The Vegetarian Diet – Can It Really Prevent Disease?

https://www.createspace.com/5519874

Is a vegetarian diet right for you? Multiple studies have shown over and over that a vegetarian diet goes along way in preventing certain chronic diseases, such as:

• Heart Disease
• Cancer
• Diverticulitis
• Type 2 Diabetes
• Hypertension
• Obesity
• Kidney Failure

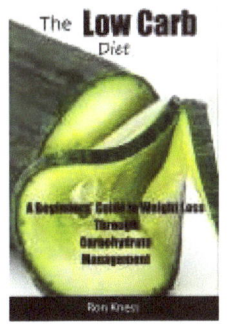

The Low Carb Diet: A Beginner's Guide to Weight Loss Through Carbohydrate Management

https://www.createspace.com/5416348

In my book "The Low-Carb Diet – A Beginners' Guide to Weight Loss Through Carbohydrate Management", I reveal a successful method of losing weight based in part on the amount and type of carbohydrates you consume.

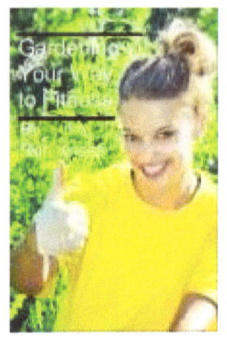

[Gardening Your Way to Fitness: The Fun Way to Get Fit and Provide Beauty and Healthful Bounty for Your Family](https://www.createspace.com/5459564)

https://www.createspace.com/5459564

The gym is a great place to stay fit during the colder seasons, but once the temperature turns warmer you want to spend more time outside. Plus, you'll have the benefit of fresh wholesome produce to enjoy by growing vegetables in your backyard garden.

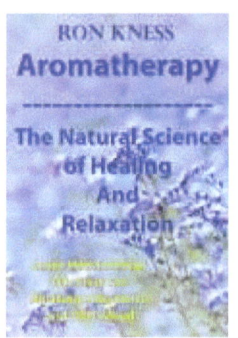

[Aromatherapy - The Science of Healing and Relaxation: Learn How Essential Oils Elicit The Relaxation Response And Alter Mood](https://www.createspace.com/5714434)

https://www.createspace.com/5714434

In my book Aromatherapy – The Science of Healing and Relaxation, we reveal the natural holistics methods you can use to heal the body from certain medical issues and to relive stress through relaxation. In particular we talk about:
• Aromatherapy - what it is and how it works

• Essential Oils – how the effects of certain aromas differs from others
• Recipes – how to make your own essential oil combinations

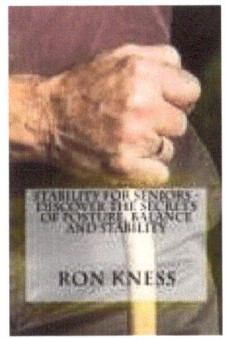

Stability for Seniors: Discover the Secrets of Posture, Balance and Stability

https://www.createspace.com/6096479

Many people sacrifice their health in pursuit of their career. They are so busy making a living that they neglect to make a life. The excuse that they do not have time to exercise is tossed about so frequently that they end up letting their health and fitness slide.

If you are not regularly active, you will have muscular atrophy over time. Your flexibility will decrease. Your core strength will diminish. As time progresses, you will be less limber and more rigid.

This is exactly how people age poorly. It's a process that has snowballed over time.

Only with regular exercise and a healthy diet can you have a body that is fit and has the ability to almost reverse aging.

If you have neglected your health for years and life seems to be a chore now because you can't get around without assistance, do not feel dejected.

You can remedy the situation. You can restore the strength, balance and stamina that you have lost. It is never too late to become what you might have been.

This guide will show you exactly what you need to do to restore your balance, strengthen your core and give you the ability to live life to its fullest. Read how …

About the Author

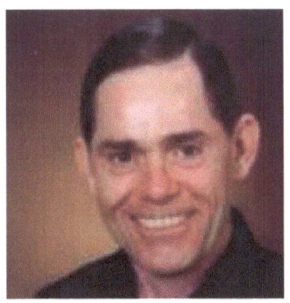 Besides my own writing, I also ghostwrite ebooks, reports, articles, blogs and do Kindle conversions for my clients on a variety of topics.

Today my wife and I live in Gold Canyon, AZ, where you'll find me happily sitting in my office typing away on my laptop as I work on my next book or ghostwriting project . . . that is if we are not traveling on a cruise ship - our new-found mode of travel.

If you like my book, please leave a review of it.